GOD WILL KEEP YOU THROUGH THE STORM

GOD

WILL KEEP YOU THROUGH THE STORM

KITA W. DAVIS

TATE PUBLISHING
AND ENTERPRISES, LLC

Published by Tate Publishing & Enterprises, LLC
127 E. Trade Center Terrace | Mustang, Oklahoma 73064 USA
1.888.361.9473 | www.tatepublishing.com

Tate Publishing is committed to excellence in the publishing industry. The company reflects the philosophy established by the founders, based on Psalm 68:11,

"The Lord gave the word and great was the company of those who published it."

Cover design by Nino Carlo Suico
Interior design by Manolito Bastasa
Author photo by Savalia Beaz

Published in the United States of America

ISBN: 978-1-62854-037-6
Self-Help / Journaling
15.06.02

To those who have or is caring for a parent with dementia or Alzheimer's disease. You have walked a path that no person should ever have to alone. You have selflessly done it for no other reason than the unconditional love that is returned to that parent when roles have been reversed.

When the battle of the disease has succumbed to death and you reach a point where you feel the pain of that loss is more than you can bear, it is at that moment that God will send a beautiful rainbow to let you know that it is him and him alone who has kept you through your storm.

To Mother

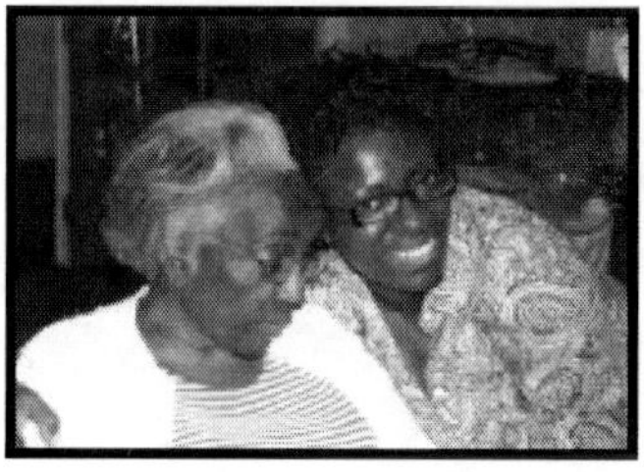

You were a mother to so many children throughout your years as a foster mother; you gave them unconditional love in so many ways. You touched the hearts and minds of these children with your dedication to their happiness. You gave them more than they could ever return; you gave them you.

ACKNOWLEDGMENTS

To my brother Minister Timothy Davis and my sister Ms. Sandra Fuqua, I love you with all my heart. We went through quite a storm together, but on the other side of it came rainbows of unconditional love and respect for one another.

To Tracy Johnson, Dr. Cynthia Jackson and Dr. Barbara Canada, your unconditional love for my family helped us to make it through a time of crisis that only God knew we could endure. Without the amazing unconditional love that you showered on my family during our time of grief, we would not have been able to make it the way that we did. Your prayers, your meals, your sacrifices, and your kindness will never be forgotten.

To my editor Ms. Renée Purdie, thank you so much. You helped turn a good book into a great book.

To the Temple Church Intercessory Prayer team and to the most awesome prayer warrior on this side of heaven, the late Mr. Terry Maurice Teasley, who went home to be with the Lord, shortly before this book was published. You held my family together with your war cries that went straight to God's ear. Thank you so much.

To my foster brothers and sisters Michael, Darlene, Galen, and Teressa, your presence meant so much to have you there with us to say good-bye to our mother. I know that she meant more to each of you than I could ever know. And last but not least, to the amazing nurses, doctors, chaplains, and social workers at Alive Hospice in Nashville, Tennessee. You made our stay unimaginable. You gave our mother and our family such great care and comfort. I cannot imagine going through the transition of death and not be in your care.

CONTENTS

FOREWORD

Every now and then in life, you are blessed to meet someone who is blessing others through their lives and their actions.

After speaking for a church conference in Maryland, a young lady stood in the line to purchase one of my books. She mentioned she was finishing her book on the challenges and blessings of being a caretaker to an elderly parent and what she learned through the process. As I listened and looked in her eyes, I knew this lady was on a mission to help others in their elderly parent journey.

When she asked me if I would consider writing a foreword for her book, I immediately remembered the moment I asked the same of Dr. Stephen Covey (*The 7 Habits of Highly Effective People*) when I was on tour with him in Australia. When I first asked, his assistant shot me down and said he didn't do forewords, but Dr. Covey looked in my eyes and saw my passion and consented. Dr. Covey's foreword ended up being one of the best I've ever seen in a book. So I, too, consented to do her foreword!

In the foreword, I want to share some ideas on how to maximize this book. First, I want you to read and reread this book and then share the book with others who are traveling this elder care journey. Although this work is a personal story, it is a road that many of us will travel! Kita is able to articulate grief, guilt, and sometimes, simply weariness for the work that is just so hard, but so much important.

Kita takes us on a journey through the life of a wonderful woman (who happens to be her mother) and how she ultimately becomes her mother's caretaker, all while managing the difficult role of being a single parent. Through it all, she displays courage and strength that will inspire you.

This is such a relevant work because the dreadful disease of dementia affects millions of people. Family and friends make the difficult decision of being caregivers without knowing the sacrifices that must be made to successfully step into that role. Many are unprepared for the emotional, physical, and mental anguish that it leaves on the caregiver. But blessings come with that burden when you change your attitude!

For anyone thinking of caring for a loved one with dementia, this is a must read! Through her selfless acts of service to her mother, Kita teaches others how "God will keep you through the storm."

—Dr. Willie Jolley, CSP, CPAE
Hall of Fame Speaker, Radio and TV
Personality, and Best-Selling Author of *A Setback Is A Setup For A Comeback*

THE CALL

The number that flashed across my caller ID was from the nursing home facility where my mother had resided since the progression of her dementia. The voice on the other end of the phone was calling to alert me that a chest X-ray was needed on my mother. "She is very congested and not very responsive," she said. "Once we have the results, we will call you back."

Normally, I would have waited until I was called with an update, but there was something different about this call that made me call back. When I called, I was told that my mother had the X-ray, and it came back clear. The nurse then proceeded to tell me that she was still lethargic. I told her that she needed to immediately send my mother to the emergency room, something I had never done before.

The nurse said that she would write the order and have her sent to the emergency room. I called my sister and brother to alert them about the day's events and request that they meet the ambulance at the hospital to see what was going on. I had moved to Tucson, Arizona, three years earlier, and it became very difficult to keep an eye on my mother's health being so far away.

I was later told by my brother that my mother had pneumonia and congestive heart failure along with her dementia/Alzheimer's disease. I was a bit perplexed as to why the earlier X-ray did not reveal this fact.

My mother was admitted to Baptist Hospital on Saturday morning December 1, 2012, and over the course of the weekend, there was very little change in her condition. I knew that something was dreadfully wrong because fear began to consume me. I felt a sense of urgency that I needed to make that five-and-a-half-hour flight back to Nashville, Tennessee, so I picked up the phone, made the reservation, and proceeded to prepare myself for the unknown.

The flight was long and quiet. It was almost as if time stood still. I was afraid because I did not know what awaited me once I arrived at my destination. When the plane landed, I headed straight to the hospital, already prepared to stay as long as I needed to, but that plan was short-lived. After only four days, my mother was sent to Alive Hospice, and it was there that she fought for the next twenty-four days. On the twenty-seventh day of December 2012 at 10:29 p.m., with friends and family by her side, she took her last and final breath.

When thou passest through the waters, I will be with thee; and through the rivers, they shall not overflow thee: when thou walkest through the fire, thou shalt not be burned; neither shall the flame kindle upon thee.

—Isaiah 43:2 (ASV)

1

THE BEGINNING OF THE END

Day 2: Sunday, December 2, 2012

When I walked into mother's hospital room and saw her, it was as if time stood still. I looked at my mother lying there with tubes up her nose and an IV stand with at least five bags of different fluids running through her veins. Her eyes were slightly open. I slowly walked up, knelt beside her bed, and whispered softly in her ear, "Mama, it's Kita, I'm here."

There were so many times as Mother grew older that this same scene would play out, time and time again. She would be brought to the emergency room, and be rehydrated, given antibiotics for an infection, released, and then sent back to the nursing home. But this time, it was different. This time, I felt that it would not be a quick trip to check on her, and before the week was over, my fears had been confirmed.

I dropped my bags in the corner of the room and prepared to hunker down for the duration of what I did not know or expect was coming. I sat there alone, in the quiet and stillness of the night, watching her breathe while waiting for her to respond to my voice. I gently rubbed her cheek with my index finger, hoping and praying that it would stimulate her to awaken, but it did not.

The nurse came in to check her vitals. I introduced myself and watched as the nurse took her pulse and checked her breathing, blood pressure, and heart rate. The nurse looked at me and said that all her vitals were normal. The questions running through my mind would have to wait until the next morning when her doctor was present.

So at the end of my first day with Mother, I stretched out on the recliner, grabbed a sweater, said a prayer, and closed my eyes for the night.

Day 3: Monday, December 3, 2012

I was awakened several times during the course of the night by nurses coming in and out of the room to turn mother and check her vitals. I managed to quickly fall back asleep but was awakened only a short time later by the sun peeking through the shades. I got up, went over to the sink and washed my face, brushed my teeth, and waited for the doctor to arrive.

Within an hour, the doctor came in with the diagnosis. "Your mother has pneumonia and is extremely dehydrated," she said. "We have also done a swallowing study on her, and she is no longer able to swallow. We are giving her glucose in her IV to provide her with limited nutrients to sustain her."

I looked at the doctor and asked a question that I did not know if I really wanted an answer to, but yet I still had to ask. "So if she cannot swallow, what does that mean?"

The doctor looked at me and said, "We will have to insert a feeding tube into her stomach in order to feed her."

Without any hesitation and clearly before I had a moment to think about it or to consult with my siblings, I said, "No! I don't want to cause my mother anymore pain."

The doctor told me that it was a simple procedure and was the only option, if I wanted my mother to live.

I was my mother's power of attorney, so that meant I had to ultimately make this difficult decision, but no matter what anyone else thought or said, it was still a decision that no one would want to make alone. I sat there quietly for a moment and then picked up the phone to call my siblings. I asked them to come to the hospital because together, we had a decision to make, and it would be that decision that would determine if mother would be able to live with a feeding tube—or die without it—because she was no longer able to swallow her food. In the end, I wish the decision had only been that simple.

Several hours passed, and my siblings finally arrived. I told them what the doctor had said, and then I started to cry. My brother immediately said, "Yes, we have to do this." I looked at my sister, and with the same passion that I held, she said no. We clearly needed more information, a better understanding of this procedure, and what, if any, complications would result from the feeding tube. My brother suggested that we call Dr. Dunn, a longtime friend of my mother, who just happened to be a gastroenterologist. So we agreed to wait until my brother spoke with Dr. Dunn to get a clearer understanding of what we clearly did not understand.

Day 4: Tuesday, December 4, 2012

There had been no change in her condition since I had arrived, so today would be the day that I started calling family members to inform them about mother's diminishing health.

After my brother consulted with Dr. Dunn about the procedure, his advice to us was instead of placing a feeding tube through her stomach, have the doctor first try the feeding tube through her nose and down her throat to see if she could even digest any form of nourishment with minimal pain. We all agreed as a family that this would be the best course of action for the time being.

2

The Reality of It All

As family members began to arrive to spend whatever time they had left with Mother, stories of her love touched us all. They each shared their fond memories of how she individually touched their lives with her heart of gold. Her hospital room, for the most part, was filled with family during the evening hours, but I longed for that quiet time that I would spend with her during the day. I explained to each family member what we knew thus far, and that we were hopeful that the procedure would be a success.

Mother had endured the devastating disease of dementia for seven long years. It had seemed like only yesterday when I walked into her nursing home room, and she did not recognize me as her daughter. This would be the first time that I felt the loss of the person I knew as my mother. I remembered thinking that to lose her physical body would be an easier loss. Maybe I thought the pain could not be as deep as the pain I felt when I looked in her eyes and realized that while she knew the familiarity of my voice, she did not know me as her daughter.

I thought back on the time several years before she had to be taken to the nursing home. It was a Saturday night. She called me because she could not get her front door unlocked. When I arrived, she was sitting in a chair by the door, fully dressed for church. I told her that it was Saturday night, and I helped her undress and put her to bed. I remembered leaving her home that night, knowing that it would not be a good idea to continue to let her live alone. I returned the next morning to check on her, and she was still sleeping. I went through her refrigerator to find her something to eat and noticed that much of the food had spoiled. I remembered thinking that she had hidden the disease well, but one of my siblings or I should have noticed something much sooner. I was saddened at the thought that my life had been so busy as a single parent that I did not notice how much my mother needed me.

Even though I was a single parent at the time, the decision was made that Mother would come to live with me and my children. I soon found out that being a caretaker and a single parent was extremely difficult. Trying to juggle getting children off to school, getting Mother dressed to go to adult day care, and then going to work was extremely tiresome. After work, I would pick Mother up from adult day care, cook dinner for the family, bathe her, and then do it all over again the next day. Eventually, after two years, it had taken its toll on my body, and Mother had gotten to the point where she did not want to get up and go to day care. I had no other choice but to leave her at home alone. I turned the television on, left her lunch, and let her know by showing her the hands on the clock what time I would return.

This scenario was short-lived. It ended when I received a call from a neighbor alerting me that she had picked up Mother not far from my house walking down a very busy street. Mother had tried to walk back to her home. It was at this point that I was forced to make the hard decision to be responsible for my mother's life—or her death.

I was told that she needed to be placed in a more skilled facility, and it was at this point that the difficult decision was made to place her into an assisted living facility.

3

A Glimmer of Hope

Day 5: Wednesday, December 5, 2012, 7:30 a.m.

The technicians came to escort Mother from her room to have the feeding tube inserted through her nose. As they rolled her down to radiology, I followed closely behind them. They told me that I could stay and watch, but I elected to go to the chapel instead. I needed some time alone to commune with God. As I sat quietly in the chapel, the tears began to flow. My heart ached with excruciating pain, the type of pain that only God could feel. As the tears fell like thick drops of rain, it felt as if I was frozen in time. When the tears finally stopped, I felt the peace of God consume me. I stood up, pulled myself together, and started the long walk back to my mother's room.

When I arrived at her door, I took a deep breath before I walked in. I looked at my mother lying there with the feeding tube up her nose and wondered if she was in any pain. After awhile, I started to notice the different sounds that she would make when she was in pain. She could not communicate with us through normal means, but after awhile, I knew when to ring the buzzer to ask for pain medication for her. Although the medicine would put her to sleep, it was comforting to know that she was not in any distress. After most of the day had passed, the nurse finally came in and poured a can of Ensure into yet another bag that would be attached to her IV stand. As I watched the milky-like substance enter through the tube, I waited and prayed that the procedure would be successful.

Later that day, the nurse came back to extract the Ensure from her stomach. This would determine how much, if any, she would be able to digest. What came out was disturbing. It did not look like the same substance that went in. I watched the nurse continue to extract what was in her stomach until it was all out. I knew that this was not a good sign. The nurse looked at me and said, “We will need to wait a little while before we try it again.”

Later that evening, my brother came to visit and brought with him one of my cousins. As our cousin knelt over her, he began to talk to her but soon started to weep. He was expressing to her how much he loved her and appreciated all that she had done for him. I went over to him, wrapped my arms around him, and told him that the best thing he could do for her was to do what she taught him to do. She taught him to love the Lord, with all his heart and soul, but somewhere along his way, he had lost sight of that.

I asked my family to gather around him. As we stood there together, we all held hands, and I began to pray for him. As difficult as the day had started, just the simple fact that it ended with us as a family gathered around my mother, in prayer for another family member would have made her rejoice. And although she was not awake, I truly felt that had she been, her words to us would have been: "Today was a good day."

The one thing that my mother was consistent about as a foster mother was to share the love of Jesus Christ. It was important to her to read stories of the Bible to the children who were in her care. After supper, she would read to them and then ask them questions to make sure that they were listening. It was her way of making sure that a seed was planted in their hearts. And no matter how long or how brief, their stay was, they would leave with an everlasting knowledge of Jesus Christ.

Train up a child in the way he should go:
and when he is old, he will not depart from it.

—Proverbs 22:6 (KJV)

4

Reality Sets In

Day 6: Thursday, December 6, 2012

During the course of the night, the nurse came in to extract more of the liquid that was in Mother's stomach. It was a greenish substance, unlike what was extracted earlier. When I asked the nurse what it was, I was not ready for the answer. Apparently, some of her vital organs had begun the process of shutting down, and her bowels had backed up into her digestive track. It also seemed that more was being extracted than went in. The nurse unhooked the liquid bag from the feeding tube in order to give mother's stomach time to digest what was already there.

Later during the day, the nurse came back and tried the feeding again. After several hours passed, the nurse came back to extract the liquid once more, but this time, nothing came up. Oh the joy that flooded my soul to know that it was going to work, and yes, Mother may have a fighting chance! But the excitement was short-lived.

To relieve myself from everything that was going on around me, I agreed to speak at a ladies' group during the afternoon. Initially, I had welcomed the idea of committing myself to something that would force me to leave the hospital, but as I was driving away, all I could think about was getting back.

I pulled up to the church in an almost-comatose state. I saw people, but I had no emotions. I ate, I laughed, I fellowshipped, but all I felt was emptiness. It was only when I got up to speak did the courage rise up in me to pull out what God had placed there for these ladies. There is something about drawing strength from God in the midst of devastating circumstances that will show you who you really are and what you are really made of.

I made it through the afternoon with the ladies but hurriedly went back to the hospital. Later during the evening, the nurse came in again to see if my mother was able to digest the last feeding of Ensure. Once again, she began to extract the liquid from my mother's stomach. The syringe began to fill with the liquid nutrients that she could not digest. I felt that this would be the last attempt to try to feed Mother because the last several attempts to feed her had failed.

5

ONE MOMENT IN TIME

Day 7: Friday December 7, 2012

I had a sleepless night as I lay in the recliner next to my mother's bed. I got up several times during the night to sing to her. She loved music. My daughter came in and put Pandora radio on Mahalia Jackson. She said, "Granny wants to listen to this!" I kindly obliged.

At some point during the night, the nurse had stopped the feeding and IV fluids. I knew in my heart what that meant, but I dared not let my mind solidify my thoughts.

The doctor came into the room and said, "Your mother has not eaten for nine days, and we have stopped giving her fluids. We are now going to send her to Alive Hospice because there is nothing more that we can do for her here."

I heard the words, and I saw the doctor's lips moving, but I could not comprehend what I was hearing. "There is nothing more that we can do for her here" was what the doctor was saying, but what I heard in my mind was, *Your mother is dying*. Suddenly, it was as if I was standing inside a bubble. I could see the doctor, but I could not move, I could not speak, and there was suddenly confusion around me. It didn't make sense. She was simply dehydrated. She had pneumonia. *All she needed was some fluids to rehydrate her, and then she could go back to the nursing home*, I could hear myself thinking, but no words were spoken. I was completely numb.

Day 8: Saturday, December 8, 2012

Four years earlier, I had volunteered at the very same Alive Hospice that my mother was being sent to. I knew that my mother would be comfortable here, and that she would be kept free from pain until it was time for her to move on to her final resting place.

I was contacted by the hospice admissions department to come and sign the paperwork needed to admit my mother to the facility. I was told that the ambulance would be at the hospital to pick her up at two thirty. While my sister and daughter waited at the hospital with my mother, I drove to Alive Hospice, signed the paperwork, and waited for her to arrive. While I sat in the office and talked with the administrator, I began to cry because of the certainty that my mother would not leave this facility the same way that she came in.

Room 188 was her room. I walked into the room, and it felt familiar to me. I did not remember the person who I had seen in it when I volunteered here, but I did remember the room. As I waited for Mother to arrive, I walked through the halls of that facility, and a great calm engulfed me.

By the time I made it all the way around the facility, I saw the ambulance approaching the door. I knew it was my mother. The ambulance attendants wheeled mother through the entrance doors, and the person at the front desk told them to go to room 188. Apparently, they had made this trip often as they knew exactly which way to go.

"One, two, three," the ambulance attendants counted as they pulled her from the gurney onto her bed. The nurses immediately surrounded her and began to check her vitals. I told them she needed something for pain as she had started to grimace and moan. The nurse brought her something and placed it in her mouth. I told the nurse that she had trouble swallowing and the IV was left in her hand in order to administer the medicine there. The next dose of medicine until the last would be given to her through the IV.

The question was asked. "Would anyone be staying with her?" I said that I would. Once again, I hunkered down in what would be my home until my mother went to be with God.

Then I heard the voice of the Lord saying,
"Whom shall I send? And who will go for us?"
And I said, "Here am I. Send me!"

—Isaiah 6:8 (NIV)

6

For Everything, There Is a Season

Day 9: Sunday, December 9, 2012

I was awakened every two hours during the night when the nurse came in to turn Mother. At every moan, I would jump up to see if she was okay. When she did that, I knew that she was in pain. The nurses came within fifteen minutes to administer morphine, and within another fifteen minutes, she would fall asleep again. The doctor came in, introduced herself, and explained that she would be examining my mother and checking her vitals.

"Her heart rate is good," the doctor said. "The pulse and bowels sounds, good. Her breathing is good, and she is resting peacefully."

I smiled as the doctor exited the room.

Next to my mother's bed was a leather recliner, and it was in this recliner that I made peace with my mother. My mother had been a foster parent for many years. It started out with just one baby, then two, then a family of four. My mother had only belonged to my brother and me, and suddenly, I had to share her with children who were not her own. As she started to show love toward them, I began to resent her. I began to see her as not a foster mother, but simply mother to each child who revolved in and out of our home. I watched her as she would get up at the crack of dawn and cook a hot breakfast for them. I watched her as she cooked dinner every night for them, and I watched her as she charged up her credit cards so that the children would have nice clothes to wear. I became angry and more resentful as her love was now extended to all those other children.

I felt betrayed by her. I felt jealous as I saw her and my father do things for one of the children who would ultimately become my adopted sister. She had separation anxiety each time she left our home to be adopted. When she first came to our home, she came to us as an abused child, and she was so very fragile. I remember looking down at her in a full body cast, wondering who could do this to a baby. I fell in love with her but became angry at her when I saw how much my parents loved her.

I eventually joined the army because I felt that my mother did not have time to be a mother to me in the most important years of my life. Looking back, it all seems so very insignificant as I realized that she loved me the best that she could. I came to terms with the fact that the children she brought into our home were also providing income for her to help raise our family.

After spending eleven years in the army, I now had two children of my own. I did not realize it then, but I had to learn a very difficult and painful lesson through my own children. I realized that I did not have the maternal love that mothers feel for their children, so I never developed the emotional attachment to my children that most mothers have. To combat that, I tried to show them love through material things. My mother raised my firstborn son while I served my country. When he was two years old, I came home from Germany to get him, and it broke her heart. When I received orders to go to Korea, once again, my mother cared for my children while I served abroad. I had been in Korea for about six months when my mother became ill. I had developed some medical problems myself from being in the military, so I elected to take a medical retirement so that I could care for my children and my mother.

My mother eventually got better, but the bond between my son and my mother had already been established. I started to understand how my mother must have felt when I bonded with my Aunt Fannie. Aunt Fannie was the caretaker who cared for me and my brother while my mother worked before she became a foster parent. She wasn't related to us, but that was what we called her, and she became like a mother to me.

Over the years, I slowly began to forgive my mom although I had no right to withdraw my love from her in the first place. She is, and was, the epitome of what love is. I remembered watching her as she read Bible stories to the children before bed. I remembered her dressing them in their Sunday's best that she had bought for them from JCPenney on Church Street. I watched as she dressed them for church every Sunday. I remember the big Sunday dinners we had as all eight of us squeezed in around our kitchen table. I remembered our traditional family Christmas dinners where the kids and I would iron the tablecloth, shine the sterling silver flatware, and wash the Christmas glasses because of the dust that had settled on them throughout the previous year. Those glasses had a special place in the brown china cabinet that stood in our dining room for many years. Memories of years past flooded my memory and began to make me smile.

That Brown China Cabinet

Renée Purdie

That brown china cabinet
Is filled with more than dust
It's filled with memories,
memories that I trust
Glass and silver curios
relics of days gone by
How I love that brown china cabinet,
Even the memories that make me sigh

My mother was diagnosed with dementia in 2006, but she had hidden it from us for some time. Looking back, I saw things that I chose to ignore because after all, she was my mother, and I had my own home and family to raise. I thought back again to that Saturday night when she called me because she could not find her house keys to unlock the deadbolt on her front door.

My brother was married with three children. My sister was married. And then there was me, divorced and raising two children alone. I had a three-bedroom home and ended up putting my mother in the master bedroom and putting a twin bed in the small dining room, which became my room.

There were times when mother would lock herself in the bathroom, fall asleep on the commode, and I would have to pry the door open to get to her. It became difficult for me to lift her in and out of the tub, and I started to suffer physically and emotionally. I was told by my doctor that the load was too heavy for me to carry alone, and for my health, I needed to look at other options to care for her. I spoke with my mother's primary care doctor, and she admitted her into the hospital in order to place her in a skilled nursing facility. I followed through with what her doctor suggested, but once she was admitted into the facility, she could not understand why I was leaving her there. She was so angry at me. I remember her saying to me that I would not treat a dog the way that I had treated her by leaving her there. I could not get that statement out of my mind, so within two weeks, I moved my mother back into my home again.

After mother wandered away from home, she was placed into assisted living, and she did very well there for a while but then after about a year, started to steadily decline. She became very depressed and incontinent. One morning, I received a call from the police department alerting me that my mother had been picked up walking down a very dangerous street at four-thirty in the morning. Apparently, she had found the one door that could be opened to the outside from her floor and exited the building. It wasn't very long after that when it was decided that she no longer fit the criteria for assisted living. It was a severe blow for both of us because the woman in the picture below is the woman I remembered: sassy, indomitable, fiercely independent. I definitely learned that apart from God who never fails and never changes, the only constant is change.

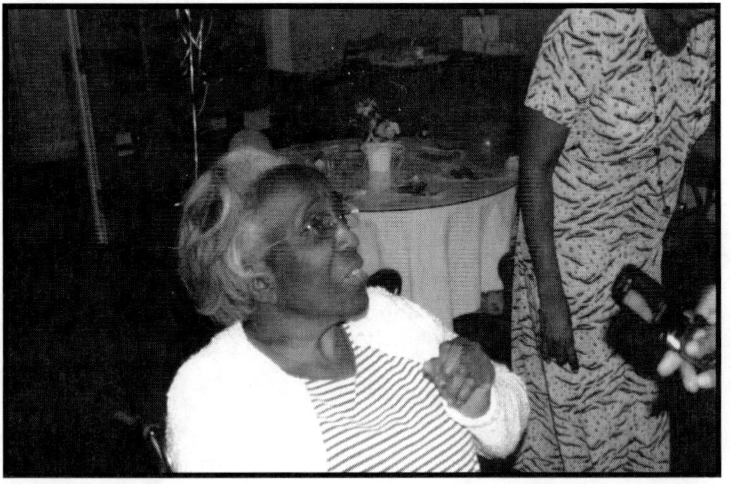

7

A Season to Cry

Day 10: Monday, December 10, 2012

The call was made to relatives out of state as well as the foster children who remained close to Mom throughout the years. They all came to say their good-byes, but it was my son who loved her most of all and found it the most difficult to let her go.

He took such good care of her after I moved to Tucson, Arizona, just three years earlier. I moved to Tucson after receiving a promotion with my job. I had raised my two children, taken care of my mother and father (deceased), so I felt it was time to take care of me. Also, I had two siblings, and it was time for them to step up to the plate and take care of her. My plan was to go there for the promotion, work really hard to get promoted again so that I could make enough money to come back home and move my mother into my home again, but this time, with the assistance of home health. God's plan for mother was not my plan, and although painful, I had to trust the plan of God—for my life as well as hers.

Once back home in Nashville, I had to face the harsh reality that my son had not spoken to me in nine months. He was angry with me for a number of reasons and chose not to be a part of my life. The entire week that she was in the hospital, he did not visit. More likely than not, it was because he knew that I was there, but once she was moved to hospice, he could not stay away.

After twelve days, I spent one night away from my mother to wash my clothes and get a good night's rest. When I entered my mother's room the next morning, there in the recliner was my son. As much as I wanted to embrace him, I simply had to wait until he was ready.

Day 11: Tuesday, December 10, 2012

It had been almost two weeks since Mom had eaten and close to seven days since she had water. All her medications had ceased, to include her blood pressure medication, her thyroid medication, and her heart medication, but yet and still all her vital signs were strong. My children, my brother, my sister, and sometimes cousins held a vigil in her room.

She was never left alone. Every time she opened her eyes, I wanted her to see me or someone whom she recognized so that she would know that she wasn't alone. I saw the toil that it was taking on my siblings and her grandchildren, but I was able to remain strong. With that said, I had my moments of sheer pain where I would rest my head on her shoulder, telling her how sorry I was and asking for her forgiveness.

I watched my brother look in her eyes and sing to her, and I watched my sister gently caressing her face and constantly asking her if she was okay. I watched the love that my son had for her as he cleaned her eyes, wiped her mouth, and gave her drops of water through a straw. He made sure that her head was always in the most comfortable position. He watched her until he fell asleep. They truly had a special bond, and she would leap and raise her body and her head when she heard his voice. The only time I saw my mother smile was when she looked at him. Yes, she loved him in a way that I never could.

I gave him time to be with her, but as he began to cry, I took him by the hand and led him outside the room. I said to him that I was very sorry, and I knew how much he loved his grandmother. I told him that I was very proud of the way that he had cared for her. I also told him that I knew he was angry with me, and that it was okay because I understood. But yet and still he was my son, and I was going to love him where he was.

8

Beauty in the Midst of Sorrow

To console those who mourn in Zion, To give them beauty for ashes, The oil of joy for mourning, The garment of praise for the spirit of heaviness; That they may be called trees of righteousness, The planting of the Lord, that He may be glorified.

—Isaiah 61:3 (NKJV)

Day 12: Wednesday, December 12, 2012

Today was very difficult. Mother needed pain meds more frequently, and she was no longer having bowel movements. She was coughing a lot and given medicine to break up the congestion in her chest. She would sleep a lot with her mouth open, and when she would open her eyes, she would look at something that no one else could see. She would try to raise her head as if she was trying to get to whatever it was that she could see. Her eyes had turned colors from dark brown to sometimes a beautiful sky blue to a jaundice yellow, and they were very glassy. Her skin was still beautiful. She didn't have one wrinkle, and it was as soft as silk. Although she was coughing more, she appeared to be more alert, but not alert to anything that I can see.

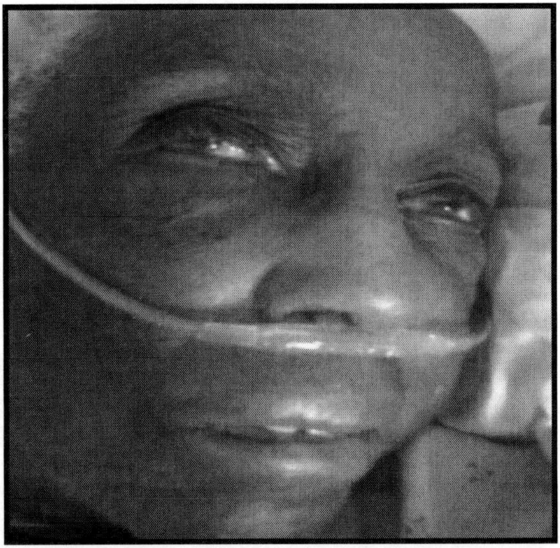

For two weeks, I had been with my mother day and night, and I was beginning to feel the emotional toll. The doctor came in, and she said after taking her vitals, "Your mother is now down to hours or days." I looked at her and just said, "Okay." The chaplain followed suit and said a prayer and made mention that she would most likely not see me the following Monday. They had given up hope, but I and the rest of my family could not. My son, her beloved grandson, had to go out of town, but before he left, he whispered to her to hold on until he returned.

9

Angels Watching Over Us

Be not forgetful to entertain strangers: for thereby some have entertained angels unawares.

—Hebrews 13:2 (KJV)

I went to sit outside Mother's room, and I saw a man whom I had watched go up and down the hall to the break room and back to the room diagonally across the hall from my mother. I decided to visit the room next door to my mother's room just to say hello to the daughter who was there with her ninety-two-year-old mother, and then there was the young pastor who was there for his forty-nine-year-old uncle who was directly across the hall from Mother.

As I returned to my seat outside of my mother's room, the wife of the father whom I watched going back and forth began to talk with me. She started telling me about her daughter who was also forty-nine. I felt compelled to ask her if I could go visit with her daughter. She said that she would like that. As I walked into the room, I was not prepared for what I saw. There laying in front of me was a beautiful angel. Her face was suffused with a radiant light, her hair was long and blond. And although she appeared to be less than ninety pounds, she was the most beautiful woman—besides my mother—whom I had ever seen. I called her Angel and asked her if I could pray for her, and she said that I could. I joined hands with her family, and I began to pray. As I finished my prayer, she also asked if she could say a prayer for me. I said yes, and she did. There is just something about knowing the Lord that connects spirits together in a supernatural way. I connected with Angel that night, and I truly believed that even though she was also soon to be with the Lord, that God still had a purpose for her. I felt that somehow her spirit connected with my mother's, and that my mother would go first and be waiting to welcome Angel to her new home in heaven.

Day 13: Thursday December 13, 2012

I could tell that my mother was in distress. She was sleeping more with her mouth open and eyes partially closed. Sleep deprivation was taking its toll on my body. Every time I heard her moan, cough, or wheeze, I would jump up to make sure that she was okay. The doctor came in again to examine her, and after the examination, the doctor looked up at me and said, "I think she is down to days or weeks." I had a small glimmer of hope, followed by an unrealistic expectation, believing that after two weeks without food or water, Mother could still continue to hold on.

I felt the strength and love of my mother being imparted into me, and even as the love we shared began to well up in me, I felt that there was no way I could continue to go on the way that I had been. I wanted to leave and not come back. I wanted to remember her alive. I felt that emotionally, I had gone as far as I could go, and I had nothing left to hold on to.

Just when I needed her, my dear friend, Barbara Canada, stopped by to take me to dinner, and it was just what I needed. She treated me to either the best steak I had ever had or maybe I was just hungry, but whatever the case, it was comfort food to my soul. My mother would have said in her hilarious humor: "I have dined sufficiently. Had I dined any better, I would have dined abundantly."

We ate, and we laughed as she allowed me the time to grieve in my own way. She let me sit quietly and say nothing while I processed what was happening around me. I did not want to go back to hospice, but I had to because I was always the strong one amongst my siblings and felt that even now, I had to continue to stay strong for them. Somehow, I had to find the strength to carry on.

10

God Does All Things Well

The nurse walked in with a big smile on her face. She had with her a hideaway bed. I had asked for one the day that I arrived, but those beds were a hot commodity. As happy as I was to get it, I knew it was only because someone had passed away. The bed would give me just enough rest to stay asleep and not wake up several times during the course of the night.

I had awaken at some point during the course of the night and decided to go for a walk. Upon returning to my mother's room, there sat my brother. He said that he would be staying the night with me. It gave me comfort because my greatest fear was to wake up alone in the room with my mother only to find her gone. Although I did not verbally tell him I needed him to stay, I think my mother knew that I needed him to stay, and he felt it from her.

Day 15: Saturday, December 15, 2012

My sister came to relieve me so that I could go to church. Church was the one place where I desperately wanted and needed to be. The service was warm and heartfelt; it was just what I needed to carry me the rest of the way.

My daughter was leaving to go back to California today. I enjoyed her being here, and I am happy that she has been afforded the opportunity to spend time with her grandmother. As she would be leaving, my son would be returning. His grandmother had done what he had asked, and that was to wait for him to return.

Two of my mother's foster children, Michael and Darlene, came to visit her today. Michael lived in Louisville, Kentucky, and Darlene still lived in Nashville. To listen as they expressed how much they loved my mother, and to hear how their lives were changed because of her, and to hear that it was because of her prayers and her teachings that shaped and molded them, made me so very proud to know that her legacy will remain and she will never be forgotten.

My son had returned from his trip to Houston, and when he walked into the room and spoke, Mother heard his voice, raised her head, and opened her eyes.

If the only joy that I ever brought to my mother's life was her grandson, then whatever problems that he and I had just didn't matter. I knew that there were many other times that I brought joy to her, but Bryan Uriah Johnson was her greatest.

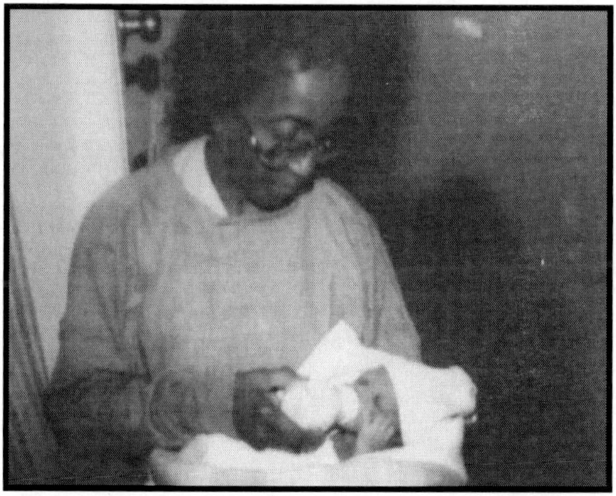

Thinking back on the time when I took her on vacation with her grandchildren to Orlando where she saw the ocean for the very first time... To remember the smile on her face at Disney, as she stood with her arms hugging Mickey Mouse... To remember her tears as I read a poem that I had written for a surprise birthday party for her...

Yes, as memories flooded back, I was reminded that there were *many* times that I brought joy to my mother.

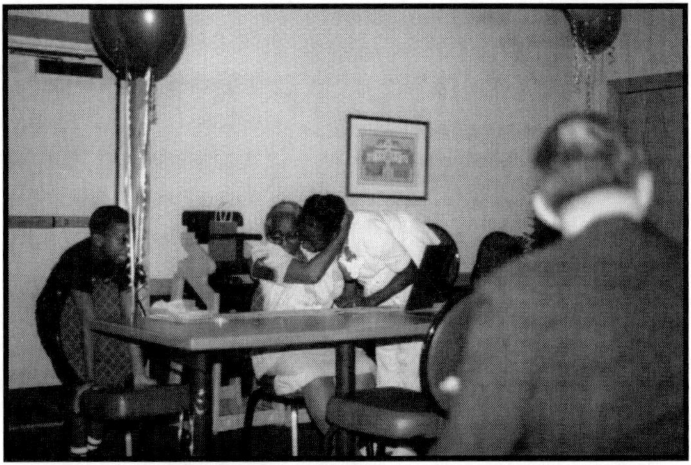

Day 16: Sunday, December 16, 2012

This was the day that I actually started writing this book. I wrote until the early hours of the morning. I *needed* to write. I needed to focus. I needed to try and give her this gift before she left me. It gave me comfort in knowing that one day, people will know her and love her even though they never met her. Some may even help carry her legacy long after she has departed this life by supporting the foundation that I will start in her honor. She loved her foster children, and one way that I can honor her name and her memory is to start a foundation that will help foster children who may have never experienced the love of a mother. The Theresa Davis Foundation will help children in foster care once they have reached the age of eighteen and are no longer eligible to be under the foster care system. The foundation will help with scholarships and job training so that those now-adult children will be afforded the same opportunity as children who grew up with their parents. I think she would be proud to know that her life and example were not in vain.

When the chaplain entered mother's room this morning, I said to her, "I bet you did not expect to see us here today." She looked at me and said, "You are right." She knelt over my mother and began to pray. I heard her tell my mother that it was okay for her to leave this life because she had lived a good life, and the evidence was her children. She said to her that we will be okay, but there are those that are waiting for her to cross over. I knew that she meant well, but I knew that when my mother was ready, no one would have to give her permission to go.

As I made that long walk from her room to the break room where there was always coffee, hot chocolate, tea, and sometimes goodies that people brought in, I saw the nephew of the man who is across from my mother's room, who happens to be the pastor of a local church.

My brother brought in meat loaf and mashed potatoes to share with the families today. I took Pastor Kerry a plate and told him to eat. There is a certain bond that takes place among people who are suffering together. Suddenly, strangers become lifetime friends. They become your confidants; they become your lifeline. We would share meals together as people brought in food in honor of their loved ones who had passed away. We would come together and talk about the lives of those we love who were about to be taken from us. We would give one another hope with just a simple smile or memory of days gone by. We would keep each other strong enough to endure another day.

When I saw Pastor Kerry sitting in the hallway with his head bowed into his cuffed hands, he had a look of exhaustion etched upon his face. I walked past him but felt the Lord leading me to go back and pray for him. I went back and sat quietly beside him. He raised his head, and I told him that the Spirit of the Lord led me to come back and pray for him. He said that he knew I was coming back. I gently took his hand and prayed that God would strengthen him.

As pastors and ministers, we give so much of ourselves. We are constantly pouring out, sometimes past the point of exhaustion. Sometimes, all it takes for us to be recharged is someone to come by and take the time to pray with us, and that was what the Lord had me do for him. I think one of the lessons in this book is to show that even in our weakness, God will strengthen us to the point of realizing that it is not about us, but it is *always* about him.

I had gotten through another day, and mother's youngest grandchild, Tiffany—my brother's daughter—would fly in today at five in the afternoon from college. I wondered if this is why she had held on. I wondered if she will now be ready to let go of this life and embrace the next.

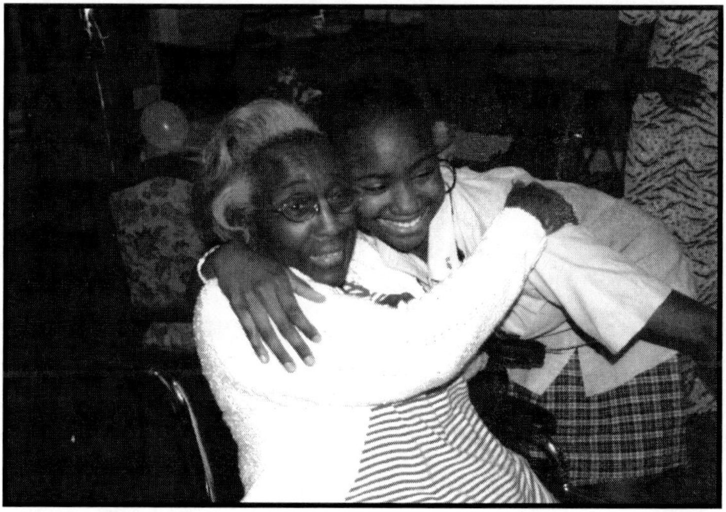

Day 17: Monday, December 17, 2012

Although I was up until two thirty in the morning writing, I awakened to a feeling of great peace. I woke up with Angel in my spirit. I got up, washed my face, brushed my teeth, and began my daily ritual. I folded up the hideaway bed, changed my clothes, brushed my hair, anointed my mother with oil, prayed for her, and then went to see Angel.

I gently knocked on the door, and her father answered with, "Good morning" as he welcomed me into her room. Angel's mother raised her head from the sofa where she was resting and smiled. I went to her, kissed her cheek, and told her that I loved her. I think Angel was posting on Facebook, so I told her that I would come back. As I was about to leave, she put away the phone and said hello. I walked over to her bed and again saw this beautiful frail body with a beautiful smile that illuminated the room. I told her that I came to see her because she was a ray of sunshine, and that I drew strength from her and needed to see her. I knelt down to embrace her and kiss her cheek, but before I could get up, I began to pray for her. I told her that she was one of God's perfect angels, and that he loved her and missed her so much that he was ready to bring her home. She embraced me, and as I arose, her father was beside me, and he embraced me as well. I have bonded with this family, and we will forever be connected.

11

FEAR

Day 18: Tuesday, December 18, 2012

Today had been the most difficult by far. I almost ordered my mother back to the hospital to be put on a ventilator. The end was drawing near, and I was devastated at the thought of losing her. She cannot stop coughing. Her lungs had begun to fill with fluid, and she had to lay with her head elevated in order to breathe. My heart felt as if someone had punched me in my chest with a boxing glove, and my tears seemed as though they would never stop falling.

A day earlier, I walked into the hall to ask the doctor if there was anything left that we could do. When she told me no, I began to weep uncontrollably. Pastor Kerry from across the hall saw me crying, and as we made eye contact, I smiled. I knew that he was going to say to me the very same things that I had spoken to him, in this same hall, almost in the exact same place. It brought comfort to my soul knowing that someone understood just how much I was hurting because they were experiencing the exact same hurt.

In speaking with him, I realized that we had quite a few things in common. We were ministers, playwrights, and directors. He had a very sweet spirit about him, and he was very easy to talk with. He shared with me how difficult his morning was as he lay in a room alone, weeping. I understood because I was just in that very same place. I am so blessed to have close friends and family near because in the midst of this pain, someone would say or do something that would allow me to break away from the pain just long enough to steal a laugh or a smile, if only for a moment.

Day 19: Wednesday; December 19, 2012

I spent most of this day reminiscing about my childhood. The nurses talked about how beautiful my mother's skin was and how loving she seemed to be. I start to laugh, and they asked me what was so funny. I said my mother was very loving, but to look at her, you would not believe that she was very comical at times. I told them some of her funny sayings:

"I'm fine as wine in the summer time."

"You can't fool a fooler."

"Flies and lies I do despise. The more you lie, the more I like flies."

I told them that it was about ten years earlier when I asked my mother, "At what age do you lose interest in sex?" My then seventy-nine-year-old mother looked at me and said, "You are going to have to ask someone older than me!"

As the day progressed, it would be a day that I needed to spend time out of my mother's room. Not only was it cold and rainy, I wanted to give my son some alone time with her. As I was sitting outside her room, the nurse practitioner walked in to visit with my mother. As she left, I asked her how she was doing. She said, "No change," the same exact words that I had heard for the last several days. She looked very bewildered though, so I asked her what was wrong. She said, "It is just that I am amazed at the strength of your mother. Because every once in a while, we will get a patient in here that defies all odds. I am simply amazed." I smiled within and said, "Yes, that's my mama!"

Later in the evening, my sister came to visit our mother. She was only in the room a short time before she came to the break room with tears in her eyes. She looked at me and said, "I can't do this tonight." I told her to sit and talk with me for a while as I did not want her to drive in that state. I said to her, that this was the closest that we have ever been. I told her that I loved her, and the strength that our mother was showing us was the strength that we had to hold on to in order to get us through this time together.

I walked her back to my mother's room to gather her things, and when I looked at my mother, I gasped. In just a few hours, she had changed. Her face was now sunken in, her mouth widely opened, and her head tilted upward. I now understood why my sister had been so upset.

I am fearful that this night may be her last day with us.

Despite the marked physical differences, Mom's vital signs are still within normal limits. Science says that the body can only go seven days without water and twenty-one days without food. My mother has gone eleven days now without water, and tomorrow, it will be the twenty-first day without food.

At eighty-nine years of age, my mother continues to do it her way. She taught me to never let people tell you what you can or cannot do, and she was showing me now that even when the doctors said that she would not make it another day, she showed them that she could.

Day 20: Thursday, December 20, 2012, 3:04 a.m.

It was going to be a very long night.

My brother, my son, and my sister-in-law have gathered around to wait. I have not been able to sleep as Mother's hands and feet have started to become cold. Her breathing was becoming shallow with each passing minute. She was not easily awakened.

My sister-in-law and my brother fell asleep, but my son and I stayed awake. I took a pair of socks from the drawer next to her bed and placed them on her feet. I began to massage her feet, almost making myself believe that I could keep her blood circulating, and that her feet would begin to warm up again.

Early the next morning, new families began to come in with their loved ones that would be admitted. Two of my closest friends Barbara and Tracy, who had been by my side almost every day, introduced themselves to the new families and offered them something to eat. I told them that we are all family here, and we all come together and share our meals.

As much as I have regretted being here, strangely I feel as if I don't want to ever leave. This had been my home for the past three weeks. The staff had become my friends, and the thought of leaving was like going up a rollercoaster, anticipating reaching the top but dreading it too because you know what is on the other side: going down. Anxiety and fear set in, and sadness was now hovering like a dark cloud over me.

6:30 a.m.

I was not sure what had awakened me, but when I opened my eyes, I saw my brother lying in the fold-out bed beside me. When I had fallen asleep, his wife was there. When I opened my eyes again, I saw my son. He was on one knee, kneeling beside his grandmother's bed, with his hand on her head.

I asked my brother what was going on, and he said that the nurse was bringing Robinul to clear up some of the congestion in her chest. Looking back, I think this was more for us than for my mother. Looking at her, I realized that this was all part of the process, and at this stage in her dying, no amount of Robinul or morphine was going to help.

I don't know which was harder, watching my mother as her breaths became more shallow and faster or watching my son, who loves his grandmother so very much. I think that it was doubly painful. I knew that she cannot go on much longer, but I had asked God not to take her yet because I knew that it would have a devastating effect on my son for years to come because this was the first of this type of grief for him.

I didn't know what to say to him. I didn't know what to say to myself. I had always been the strong one. I had always been the one to take care of everything. Did I have any regrets? Was there anything that I could have done differently? These are all questions that I can look back on now and say, "Yes!" I regret that I spent so much time selfishly thinking of only myself when I knew she needed me. I regret other things that only I would have to come to terms with. But with the realization that, yes, there are many things that I could have done differently, there is also the sure and certain knowledge that I don't think there is one person who would not also say the same in this type of situation.

Did I give up on her and just settle for what the doctor said? No! I consulted with my family, and we made decisions as a family. Looking back, would I have still gone to Tucson? Yes! There were two other siblings that could step up to the plate and care for our mother in my absence. I cannot speak for them as they will have to answer this question for themselves.

All I know was that right now, in this very moment in time, it is my writing that keeps me going. I know that just down the hall was my mother who could possibly be taking her last breath. Did I want to be there? No, I didn't. The pain of watching my mother and the pain of watching my son was too much for me to bare.

I had watched her these past twenty days defying all odds. I had developed deeper relationships with my siblings. I had experienced true, deep, abiding friendships from some of my closest friends who have been here for me in ways that they just did not have to be. They have taken care of not only me but my family as well. I had seen the outpouring of love for Mom from other family members, near and far. I had seen children whom are not of her own body but of her spirit come by to be by her side in these—her last days.

So many wonderful memories of my mother were flashing through my mind, and I wondered what God was doing in her at this moment. I wondered if her life was playing back for her. I wondered if she could see those who have gone before her standing at those Pearly Gates waiting for her. A smile had just appeared on my face as I thought about seeing her again. Will she be waiting there for me? Yes. I know that she will.

11:15 a.m.

I longed to fall asleep, if only for a little while. I went over to my mother to see how she was doing.

Remarkably, she didn't appear to be in the same distress as she was several hours ago. Her breathing had somewhat calmed down, and her feet were no longer cold. I thought I heard her snoring. Yes, she was peacefully sleeping again.

The only thing that concerned me now was that her tongue was hard and almost stuck in one place. I was sure this was making it difficult for her to get air as she was breathing through her mouth consistently now. I would get up now, take a shower, and begin my daily routine.

1:00 p.m.

The nurse practitioner came by the room to see how Mother was doing. I pointed out my mother's tongue to her. Apparently, the Robinul that they were giving her to dry up the mucus in her chest causes everything to dry up. She said that it would be okay to wet her tongue with the solution that they had given her for mouth care. So I took the long stick that had a little green sponge on the tip, dipped it in water, and began to lubricate her mouth. At first, it was difficult to get her to keep her mouth open as it appeared to be a normal reflex to bite down, but as I jiggled the sponge to pry it from the grip of her teeth, she opened her mouth. As the wet liquid began to saturate her dry mouth, her tongue became relaxed, and I was able to fully lubricate and soften the tissues in her mouth.

3:00 p.m.

I finally felt comfortable enough to leave my mother's bedside and take some time out for myself. I grabbed my friend who had been with me day and night and treated us to my favorite nail salon and got a signature manicure and pedicure. As the massage chair that I was sitting in began to knead the tightness in my back, I began to relax. Although the time I spent there was relaxing, my mind was still on my mother, but since I was in the neighborhood, I took the time to grab a bite to eat at one of my favorite restaurants.

We made it back to hospice around seven. My mother was resting quietly, and the rest of the night was quiet as well. Around ten, I decided to retreat to the break room for a while.

My favorite nurse came in and knelt down beside the chair next to me. She said, "I just want you to know that your mother has not passed urine in about twenty-four hours, so her kidneys are shutting down.

I looked at her and smiled. "Okay."

The nurse said, "I know how upset you were last night, and I just want you to be ready."

Ready? A week ago, the chaplain and the nurse practitioner did not expect her to live through the weekend, and here it is a week later, and she is still here. No one is going to tell my mother when she is going to leave this earth, not even me. She will do it her way!

Day 21: Friday, December 21, 2012

Today started out being a great day. I felt a peace that I had not felt before; so much so that I went to get a facial at Élan Skin Care. I walked into the salon with my friend Barbara who was still with me from the day before. The guy behind the counter said, "Hello, Ms. Davis, it has been some time since you have been in." I said to him that I had moved to Tucson, Arizona, and I was back because my mother was in hospice, and I came to spend her last days with her. He said how sorry he was. I filled out the paperwork and gave it back to the person behind the desk.

I was called to the back to begin my relaxing facial, and it was at that point that I realized just how exhausted I was. I kept hearing myself snoring as I kept falling asleep. It was much-needed sleep, and I longed for it to never to end.

"Okay." I heard the aesthetician say as he placed a mirror in front of my face.

What a beautiful glow, I thought.

I got up and proceeded to the counter to pay for my very expensive facial, which I felt that I was more than deserving of. As I waited for the person behind the counter to give me the total amount for my facial, he said something to me that almost made me collapse in gratitude. "This one is on us!" My God! I could not believe what just happened. As I began to cry, he came from behind the counter, hugged me, and said, "You deserve it." I knew that this was a gift from God.

12

A Turn of Events

As beautiful as the day had started, it ended just as ugly. As I was cleaning out my mother's mouth, my son left the room abruptly. I turned around and asked my friend who was still with me, "Where did he go?" She said that he had stormed out of the room. I stopped what I was doing and went after him to see what was going on. As I approached him in the break room, I asked him what was wrong. He said, "I just feel like she would not want people picking in her mouth, and all the people that have been in and out, talking loud, and watching movies should be quiet." I said that I could understand how he would feel that way. He proceeded to tell me that I shouldn't be trying to tell him anything about his father because I had messed up his lineage. Now this completely caught me off guard.

Earlier during the week, I had tried to make peace with him by giving him some information about his father as

I knew he had questions from conversations that I had with my brother. My son was conceived out of a deceptive situation. It was 1984, the year that I had joined the military. My first duty station was Ft. Sill, Oklahoma, and it was there that I met my son's father. He was a drill sergeant. He approached me in the mess hall where I was having lunch, and I just melted at the sight of this gorgeous man standing before me. He introduced himself, and we exchanged numbers. We began seeing each other frequently, and on my birthday, February 3, 1985, I found out that I was pregnant.

Once the baby's father found out, it wasn't very long after that that I received a much-unexpected call—from his wife. Yes, he was married and never told me. The child who I was carrying suddenly became a child who only I wanted to have. Devastated by this unexpected news and being offered money to terminate my pregnancy was more than I wanted to think about. The thought of terminating the life that was growing inside me, my very first child, I could not do it. During this time, I met another man who ultimately became my husband while I was pregnant. You have to be very careful of emotional decisions because those very decisions can and will come back to help you or haunt you.

My new husband wanted to take full parental rights over the child growing inside me. Right after my son was born, my then-husband called from Istanbul, Turkey, where he was stationed and asked me to name the newborn after him, which I did gladly.

Several years later, we divorced. He remarried and no longer wanted the responsibility of a child who was *now* not his own. For him to do that to an innocent child would later have consequences that only I would have to suffer.

So now, I was standing in front of this now–twenty-seven-year-old man, trying to defend myself while protecting him from the ugly truth about his father. Listening to these ugly accusations coming from my son's mouth while at the same time grieving for my dying mother now turned my feelings from concern to anger. As we walked back into my mother's room, I was suddenly filled with so much rage that I felt I was about to burst.

I called for my son to come back outside the room so I could tell him the entire truth as I was exhausted from taking the blame and the constant disrespect from my son when he had no idea of what the actual truth was. As he stepped out of the room, I began to tell him what he did not want to hear, so he turned around to go back in to my mother's room. I followed in pursuit to make him hear the truth. As the situation began to escalate, my brother looked up from where he was sitting beside my mother's bed and said, "Take it out of the room." My son would not budge, so I started to tell him the ugly truth. Before I could get another word out of my mouth, my son grabbed me with all of his might and carried me out of the room. I was screaming and struggling for him to put me down, and suddenly, this sacred place was now filled with anger and confusion. As I struggled to get free from him, I turned in haste and ended up slapping him and knocking his glasses off his face. The next thing I knew, I was back in my mother's room crying hysterically, and the family from across the hall from my mother's room came to offer prayer for our family.

As things quieted down, the room was suddenly empty. It was just me and my mother. I heard a quiet knock on the door, and as I got up to answer, I felt the pain in my side and my arms where my son had roughed me up. I opened the door and was shocked to see that my son had called the police. From working at the District Attorney's office in the Domestic Violence unit, I knew that this situation had now turned serious. My son actually hated me so much that he wanted me arrested. He told the police officer that I had slapped him, but what he failed to tell them was that he assaulted me first by putting his hands on me to remove me from my mother's room. As the officer listened to my side of the story and because my son had put his hands on me first, I was asked if I wanted to file assault charges against him. Even though my body had begun to bruise and ache with pain, I said no. I knew that if I showed the officer my bruising, they would take my son to jail.

As the officers questioned my family members who had witnessed the altercation, I went back and sat quietly beside my mother and began to weep. My son came back into the room, collected his things, kissed my mother, and left. At that point, I realized that for the past week, I had been tiptoeing around my son and catering to his emotions rather than my own. I realized that once he left, I was free to grieve my way. So as I lay my head on my mother's bed, the floodgates of tears that had been stored up in all the emotions that I was trying not to feel came bursting out. I cried until my eyes were so swollen that all I could do was fall asleep.

Day 22: Saturday, December 22, 2012

As I awakened this morning, my body was in such pain that it was difficult for me to move. My brother and my friend Barbara who was still staying with me both recommended that I go to the emergency room. I told them that if I went and told them what happened, by law, they would have to file a police report. I did not want to go through that, so I decided to just take a pain pill and simply rest.

As family members of those who had passed in previous years began to bring in food in memory of their loved ones, I gathered enough strength to grab a bite and do some laundry. The father and mother of Angel saw me in the hall. We gave each other a hug, and her father gave me a gentle kiss on my check and said, "I love you."

As the day progressed, Mother's breathing became very shallow again. She appeared to be in distress, and it seemed as if this day would be her last.

I called my sister and told her that she needed to come. When she arrived, she ran to my mother's side and began to cry. I had been very concerned about my sister because she had not cried at all. Every time, I tried to get her to talk or asked the nurse or chaplain to talk with her. All she would say is that she was okay. Several times, when I was expressing love for my mother, she would run from the room. Other times, she would wipe a single tear from her eye. As she now wept in despair, she called her ex-husband, and he called my mother's pastor and others from her church.

Day 23: Sunday, December 23, 2012

Although by this time my mother had a very low heart rate, she took a large breath, and then the sound that came out, I don't think that I will ever forget it. They call it the death rattle. From what I understand, it is the last sound and the last breath that comes from the body before it dies. As my mother took a deep breath and this sound came from her mouth, my sister ran from the room. I looked at my mother, waiting for her to stop breathing, but she didn't. She continued to take breath after breath after breath. Once again, my mother had cheated death.

I held on tight to my mother's hand and then went outside to comfort my sister and tell her that mother was still with us. She came back into the room and lay in the very place that I had lain the night before.

Today was very long and heart-wrenching, a day that did not turn out the way that death had planned, but a day that was filled with God's grace that kept our mother with us for yet another day.

At the end of the day, my body still hurt from the altercation with my son, so I decided to go to the emergency room. Once there, I told them that I had had a problem with my son, and my ribs had gotten bruised. Thankfully, they did not press with questions. I was there in the emergency room until four in the morning and returned to hospice with some much-needed pain pills.

I went to the break room and grabbed a cup of hot chocolate, and there, I met a nurse who gave me more wisdom in thirty minutes than I had received in four weeks. He was an older gentleman who looked to be close to seventy years of age. I told him the story of my mother and how she still continued to fight after twenty-three days with no food or water. I told him that because she continued to fight, I felt like maybe it was me who had given up on her, and it was me who had made the wrong decision to allow her to come here. He looked at me and reminded me that her body no longer tolerated swallowing, and that the attempts to feed her had failed, so it was not my fault because it was her body that had determined it was time to rest. I had not looked at it that way, but what a blessing the encounter was. I will forever be grateful that he took the time to just sit with me and talk.

13

A Season to Smile

Day 24: Monday, December 24, 2012

Today was Christmas Eve, and three weeks ago, I honestly believed that I would be spending this day, the next, and all others without my mother. I knelt right next to my mother's ear and talked about all the Christmas Eves we spent preparing for her annual Christmas dinner. I talked about the turkey and the dressing that she would be preparing, the homemade rolls that we would be waiting for to rise. And then there was the sweet potato casserole with the marshmallows on top that my brother always managed to pick off and eat. I talked about how elegant the table would look, with the freshly starched and pressed tablecloth and her very best china. I promised her that I would continue this tradition in honor of her memory.

At shift change, once again, the nurses and nurse technicians came back with awe in their eyes to see that, yes, my mother was yet still alive. The looks on their faces were priceless.

Day 25: Christmas Day, Tuesday, December 25, 2012

Waking up on this Christmas morning with my mother was the best Christmas that I have had in such a very long time. No Christmas tree, no presents, no children running through the house, no Christmas dinner with fine china, just my mother in her hospital bed, my brother in the recliner, and me in the hideaway bed pulled next to the window.

The nurse came in to bathe mother, and I helped her. She asked me if I wanted her to put lotion on my mother, and I told her no. I wanted to rub her in the anointing oil that had been brought for her from my intercessory prayer group.

As I rubbed the oil on my mother's body, I prayed. I asked God to heal her from the crown of her head to the soles of her feet. I asked God to breathe new life into her failing lungs, and I reminded God that he is a God of miracles, and that my mother was a miracle because she is still here.

I didn't know how much longer my mother would be with us. I only knew that as each day passed, I found more of myself in her. Her strength became my strength, her fight became my fight, and as I looked at her, I wondered what it was that she was holding on to. What was keeping her here on this earth when there is so much love and joy waiting for her on the other side of this life?

Even though I prayed and asked God to leave her here and even though I knew there were many other people who were praying for God to heal her and keep her here, I knew that God's plan was even bigger than whatever prayers were prayed. I also knew that God was working every day through my mother. Because I was here in this place, I had been able to witness to those who were lost. I had been able to pray for those who had stopped believing.

I was able to speak life to a young nurse after she saw me anoint my mother with oil. She came to me with child-like faith and asked if it was okay to ask God questions. I wrapped my arms around her and said, "Yes, you can ask God whatever you would like, and no matter what it is, he is faithful and just to answer. He is our Father, and he will hear us every time we call." I told her she should talk to him as if he were standing there next to her because he is. I told her I knew that because his Word tells us that he will never leave us or forsake us. She understood and hugged me. I prayed for this young nurse, and she thanked me and went on about her day.

Day 26: Wednesday, December 26, 2012

Today was a very sad day. I saw the young man from the military whom I had just spoken with on Friday about his grandmother walking down the hall very quietly. This morning, his grandmother closed her eyes for the very last time. He had spoken to me about his mother and how he had so many problems with her. I related to him because I am going through the same thing with my son not for the same reasons but the same thing. I explained to him that no matter the hurt, disappointment, or despair his mother had caused, she is still his mother, and one day, it may be her there on her deathbed. I didn't know how that reunion went with his mother. I did not have time to ask because today was the day that he and his family left hospice. No good-byes were said, only a nod of the head and a smile.

As evening approached, the family across the hall whom my family had grown so close to, the family whom had become my family during the many nights and early mornings that we spent talking and laughing together, the many meals that we shared, and the many nights we spent talking about our loved ones had come to an end. Darryl Norwood had passed away at 1:44 p.m., Wednesday, December 26, 2012.

14

A Season to Die

Day 27: Thursday, December 27, 2012

I was very restless during the course of the night. I found myself up at four o'clock in the morning, walking the halls not wanting to watch my mother struggling to breathe. The nurse came over to suction the phlegm from her throat. This provided her with a little relief. I looked at my mother slowly slipping away and knew that it was only a matter of time.

I found peace by going over to Angel's room to visit with her. Deep within myself, I felt that this young lady, who was only forty-nine years old and lit up her room with the glow of the Lord, was an angel in the flesh sent here by God to watch over my mother. I felt that their impending deaths, Angel and my mother, would be closely tied together.

I called my sister and told her to come. My sister was the one child that she adopted, the one child that she just could not let go. I love her so much. It was almost as if she came straight from my mother's womb. I knew that my sister was hurting more than she said and more than she showed, but I also knew she was right where she needed to be, safely laying next to our mother for what would be her final hours.

As I watched her tucked away in the safety of mother's bed, all I can do was sit here and write for whatever time remains. Mother's head was slightly tilted backward, with her mouth widely opened. It has been said that the spirit leaves through the mouth, and the reason why people die with their mouths open. I don't know how true this is, but I guess it makes sense.

The minutes have now turned into hours, and as time passes, visitors come in to say their final good-byes.

It was now eight hours later, and my mother was still somewhat with us. The doctor said that she was unconscious but can still hear us, so I told her again how much I loved her and how thankful I was that God gave her to me. I was thankful for all the wonderful lessons of unselfish love she taught me, and I prayed that I could be half the woman that she was to this world.

As I sat and watched how careful my sister was with our mother, I realized just how much she loved her. While laying on our mother's shoulder, she quickly drifted off to sleep.

The nurses returned to check her vitals and let us know that they could not find a pulse. She was still breathing, but her breathing was very shallow.

I told my sister that I needed to leave to do a bit of shopping, but I just needed to get some air. I could not sit there and do nothing to help her. As I was walking outside to get into the car, my dear friend Barbara, who had been there for me and my family throughout this journey, had come to sit with us again. I told her that I needed to leave for a little bit, and she invited me to just get into her car, and she would drive. I kindly obliged. We were gone for a couple hours, and when we returned, my other girl friend Tracy, and my sister's ex-husband had come.

I needed to keep busy as mother's breathing had gotten very heavy and very short. I called my friend Tracy into the bathroom of Mother's room and began to give her a facial. Every time she thought I was finished, I would find something else to do. When I looked at her face and realized there was nothing more I could do to her, as she patiently sat there while I practically bruised her face, I finally had to face the fact that it was time to face what was destined to happen.

My brother had turned the television off, and my sister was there, still in bed next to Mother. My brother was sitting on the other side of her, and I sat down at her feet. I looked at my mother and began to rub her legs because her feet had grown cold again. I irrationally thought that I could get the circulation moving again, and the blood would begin to flow to her heart. I began to weep with agony as I realized how futile my efforts were.

Not more than a few minutes went by when my brother said, "Kita, she is looking at you." I raised my head and looked into her eyes one last time. I jumped up, ran to the side of the bed that my brother was on, and rested my head on her stomach.

I heard my brother say, "She's gone."

I screamed, "No, she can't be." I looked at my mother, alive, one last time, and then she took her very last breath.

The nurse came in and listened for a heartbeat. There was none.

"10:29," I heard her say.

Thursday, 10:29 p.m., December 27, 2012 was the day, hour, and minute that my mother's life ended. From that second, everything seemed to move in slow motion. My sister continued to lay in bed with her. I continued to lay my head on her stomach and held her for what seemed like hours, but only minutes passed us by. I heard the nurse say, "We need to clean her up, and then you can come back into the room and spend time with her."

We all went outside the room. I ran to the room where Angel was. Her father met me at the door and hugged me. He looked into my eyes and told me how sorry he was. Angel's mother was lying down. I knelt down next to her, hugged her, and kissed her check. She spoke words to my spirit and to my heart that I will forever be grateful for. This family had become my family. Their daughter had become an angel of love to me, and I loved them so much.

My family went into the break room and talked and waited until we could go back into the room. As we walked into the room, it was very cold. My mother's upper body was still somewhat warm. All I remember was holding her and screaming, "Jesus, help me." It was at that time that I knew it was him and him alone that could heal the hurt that I was feeling deep within my soul. I sat down beside my mother, wrapped my arms around her, and just sat quietly there until I could let go. I felt comforted holding her, something I could not do while she was lying in that very same bed dying as each day passed. Looking back, I don't know why I couldn't. I just know that I didn't. But when I did, it was like it was just her and I in this world alone, if only for that moment. I knew that this would be the last time I would feel the softness and warmth of my mother's body, and I did not want that moment to end. After about twenty minutes, I was able to let her go and leave the room that had been my home for the past twenty-two days.

We arrived at my sister's home around two o'clock in the morning. I was physically and mentally exhausted. My sister left to go spend time with her boyfriend, and I was left alone in her apartment. For the first time in twenty-seven days, I quickly fell asleep.

The next morning when I awakened, I could not move. My body ached from head to toe so I just stayed there until I was able to drift back to sleep. When I awakened the next time, I looked at the clock. It was two o'clock in the afternoon, and although I had slept most of the day away, it still wasn't enough. I felt numb and empty, and all I wanted to do was sleep.

I looked at my phone, and I had many missed calls, but not once did I even hear my phone ring. I reached over to place my phone back on the nightstand, and it began to ring. I did not want to answer it, but I knew I had to.

Friends and family called, but they really did not know what to say. No one really knows what to say unless they have experienced this type of grief, and even then, it seems like the words are floating, not really sinking in, or I was just not able to feel the emotions behind the sentiments that were being expressed.

I felt drained and at a place where I just did not know what to do. For the past twenty-seven days, I lay next to my mother night and day, watching her slipping away. I took care of her the best I could, and now she was no longer here. What should I do? What should I say? And where should I go? All I knew was that I could only think past the next second, and that was what I did. I took one minute, one hour, and one day at a time.

The next few days were very difficult. My sister was not able to help me shop for Mother's burial clothes or help make arrangements. My brother ended up in the hospital with an irregular heartbeat from grief, guilt, and way too much caffeine. While he was in the hospital and my sister was not able to get out of bed, I stood strong as I had done so many times before and took care of everything.

My mother was dressed in a beautiful white linen suit with crystal and pearl buttons, crystal and pearl earrings, and yes, her Sunday hat. My mother had never entered a church without her hat, and this would be no exception.

Mother looked beautiful; so much so that the oldest member of her church called the deacon over to her casket and made it known that when it was her time, she wanted to look just like my mother.

Her service was a celebration of her life. She was celebrated by her family, her friends, and even some of her former foster children. The order of service was memories of her and her many funny sayings that always made us laugh. Once at the burial site, we further celebrated her life by releasing four beautiful white doves. There was something about watching the doves being released that brought comfort to me and my siblings. We watched the doves for about ten minutes as they flew in circles around the cemetery. We slowly piled back into the limo and returned to the church for the repast.

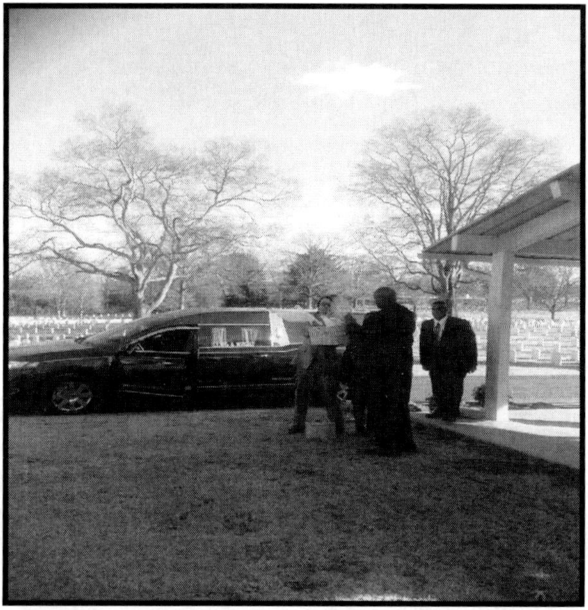

While sitting with family and friends after such an emotional morning and trying to find the right words to say, you actually end up talking "much to do about nothing." You pretend to laugh at jokes, but you only know they are jokes because the person that you are looking at is laughing. You see their lips moving. You hear the voices around you, but the only sound that is loud and clear is the sound of your heart beating through your chest.

With each heartbeat, I thought of my son who did not attend his grandmother's funeral. With each heartbeat, I thought about my daughter who did not attend either, but I also had no idea why I could not reach her. But most assuredly, I had to face the reality of my life and its impending future, returning to a place where I would be forced to deal with the past thirty days of my life. Alone—no family, no friends, no one—just me in the desert, left to deal with whatever was to come, and that whatever was more than I could have ever imagined or prepared myself for.

15

THE AFTERMATH

It is now almost seven months after the death of my mother. Never would I have imagined in my wildest nightmares that one person could endure such heartache, loss, grief, abandonment, and agonizing pain at the same time. And I never would have imagined that the person experiencing it would be me.

The series of events that happened after the death of my mother was more than enough to make anyone pack up, crawl under a rock, and die. This was how I felt almost every single day since leaving Nashville and returning to my life in Tucson, Arizona. There were very few people who knew the true extent of all that I had endured, and only God knew how many nights I put my head on my pillow, not knowing if it would be my last.

I was always the strong one. I was always the one whom the family depended upon. I was always the one who took care of our parents, who arranged the celebrations, and even after the death of my mother, I was the one who had to remain strong while making sure the arrangements were made and her home-going celebration was one that would have made her proud.

When I returned to Tucson after the funeral, not only had I spent the past month at my mother's bedside until she passed from this life, I endured a physical attack from my son and abandonment by my daughter without as much as a reason why. My brother ended up in the hospital a day after my mother died, and my sister could not emotionally be there for anyone. Through it all, I stood strong, returned to Tucson, and went back to work—and ultimately fell apart.

I began to have a series of anxiety attacks that left me clinging to my chest on the floor waiting to die. Every day that I went to work was filled with anxiety attacks, tears, and time looking for an empty office where I could find complete silence and solitude because noise was too much for me to bear.

It was not the fact that my coworkers had little regard for the pain I was feeling by having conversations about their mothers and the wonderful times they were having. I think it was more the fact that my coworkers would talk about their children and their wonderful lives, while mine was on the verge of collapse.

Eventually, the emotional grief and mental anguish took its toll on me. I had a nervous breakdown in the parking lot of my office and was taken to the hospital by my supervisor and a coworker. I stayed in the hospital for a couple days and was placed on antidepressants and anxiety medications. I was released but three days later was readmitted.

When I was too weak to stand, too weak to think, too weak to cry, and too weak to pray, I found enough courage to ask others to pray for me, and it was those prayers that gave me the strength to fight.

On June 1, 2013, I moved to Washington, DC, where God has blessed me with an amazing new job and an amazing new life. In between the transition from Tucson to Washington, DC, I returned to Nashville to try and grasp onto anything that was familiar and onto the one thing that I thought I could depend upon. It was that one thing where I thought I could find love. It was that one thing where I thought I could find strength, but it was that one thing that ultimately almost killed me.

A web of deception and lies was all that it took to rekindle the recent emotional trauma that was still well and alive within me. It was a Tuesday night when I awakened gasping and panting for air. I jumped up, ran to the bathroom, and realized that I could not breathe. I felt that I was dying, and I think in fact that I was. The heart that God gave me to love, the heart that God created to love others had taken as much as it could take, and I felt the life leaving my body as I lay back on my bed and fell back asleep.

I woke up the next morning still very short of breath, so I drove myself to the emergency room. I was admitted and for two days went through a series of CAT scans, ultrasounds, and blood work to figure out what was causing my heart to function improperly. The test came back abnormal on the first day and returned back to normal on the next. Upon admittance, the diagnosis was a mild heart attack, and upon discharge, it was noted that what I had was caused by anxiety and stress. I realized then that sometimes, you have to cut off the people in your life who would take the love that you have for them and intentionally inflict emotional pain and grief upon your life. Sometimes, you have to cut off that thing that will ultimately kill you, if you allow it to. It will try to kill your joy. It will lie to you. It will beat you down until you have no breath left in your body. Sometimes, the things that you love the most are the very things that will hurt you the most. As difficult as it is, it is those things that you have to let go and allow God to fix them. When we go through the storms of life, we are always looking for a life raft or shelter, but some storms are necessary because they will cause you to grow physically and emotionally. Some storms are necessary to clear the turmoil from your life, and some storms are allowed to happen so that you are forced to take your hands off in order for God to put his hands on and do the work that is needed to be done.

After some storms, there are beautiful rainbows that God will allow to cover you with light, love, and cascading color. After some storms, there will still be torrential downpours that end in a hurricane with massive destruction on every shore. But whatever storms that God sees fit for you to go through in your life, know this one thing: it is God and God alone who will keep you through the storm.

After two and a half years and the conclusion of this book, I have not had contact with my son, but the relationship between me and my daughter has been rekindled. I am still praying that God will work a miracle with my son, but while waiting for that storm to end, I am still trusting and depending that God will continue to keep me and carry me, until this storm has passed.

AFTERWORD

On the first year anniversary of my mother's death, I took a trip to Jamaica to finish the final edit before sending the manuscript for publication. On the morning that I was leaving, I completed the book. I put the book down, looked up, and saw a rainbow. I picked up my iPad and took a picture. I put the iPad down, looked up, and the rainbow was gone. I knew then that God had sent a rainbow just for me, to let me know that my storm had passed.

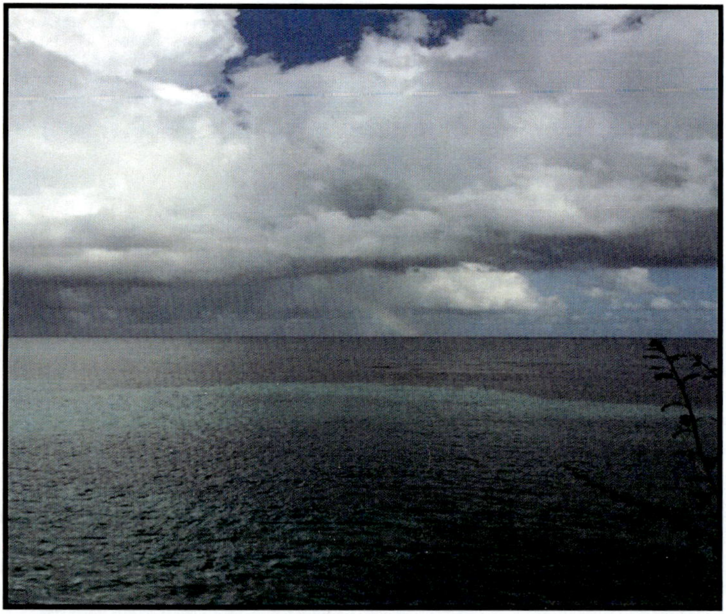

This is a sad story of the death of Rita's mom but mostly her estranged son.

Rita
703 640-4250